Essential

How to Effectively Use the Right Essential Oils to Confuse and Kill Cancer Cells

Book 1

Nancy Dennett Ducharme

Copyright © 2015 – Nancy Dennett Ducharme – All rights reserved.

No part of this publication may be reproduced, distributed, or transmitted in any form or by any means, including photocopying, recording, or other electronic or mechanical methods, without the prior written permission of the author, except in the case of brief quotations embodied in critical reviews and certain other noncommercial uses permitted by copyright law.

ISBN-13: 978-1519240538
ISBN-10: 1519240538

Photo Credits for Cover Images:

Image (cancer) ID: 10074391 courtesy of: [dream designs] at http://www.freedigitalphotos.net/images/Diseases_and_other_m_g287-Cancer_Cell_p74391.html

Image (stethoscope) ID: 100117635 courtesy of: [winnond] at http://www.freedigitalphotos.net/images/Pills_and_drugs_g279-Fish_Oil_And_Stethoscope_p117635.html

Image (rose) ID: 100188692 courtesy of: [praisaeng at http://www.freedigitalphotos.net/images/essential-rose-oils-photo-p188692

Image (pestle) ID: 100111480 courtesy of: [lemonade] at http://www.freedigitalphotos.net/images/Medical_equipment_g280-Mortar_And_Pestle_With_Herbs_With_A_Glass_Of_Alternative_Fuel_p111480.html

Disclaimer

The information in this book has not been evaluated by the Food and Drug Administration and is not intended to diagnose, treat, cure, or prevent any disease. Please consult your physician or health care provider before using any supplements.

Nancy Dennett Ducharme

Table of Contents

Disclaimer 3

Introduction 7

Chapter 1 - Blind-sided 9

Chapter 2 - Fight with Everything You've Got 13

Chapter 3 - The Cancer-Killing Power of Essential Oils 15

Chapter 4 - The Reset Button: Two Key Compounds That Create a One-Two Punch Against Cancer 19

Chapter 5 - How to Use Essential Oils Effectively 25

Chapter 6 - Remission 39

References 43

Introduction

One in three women will be diagnosed with some form of cancer in their lifetime. If you're a man, your odds have increased to a one in two chance – literally a coin toss.

Putting cancer into remission is a soul-searching, gut-wrenching, and sometimes mind-boggling journey. However, the toughest challenge I see today is not only putting cancer into remission, but **keeping** it in remission where it belongs.

Often, cancer does come back – stronger, faster, and more resistant to drugs than before. It learns to adapt.

This book will prepare you and your loved ones to fight with an advantage using some of the most powerful cancer-killing adaptogens known to man and increase the odds of beating cancer for good. In the following pages, you will learn:

- **How to use the right essential oils, in addition to your doctor's plan, to kill cancer cells faster and make your body an inhospitable place for cancer to thrive**
- Which two plant compounds **must** be used together to create a **one-two punch** to boost cancer cell death
- **Which specific essential oils to use for each type of cancer.**
- **How to apply and how to ingest these essential oils** – how much and how often.
- **How to use essential oils to assist in pain relief.**

And much more.

Let's get started.

Chapter One
Blind-sided

I will never forget the day I found out my brother had cancer.

I was in the ladies' room at my husband's office when I heard the tap on the door. "Hey, your mom's on the phone." Jeff said from behind the closed door.

"Okay, tell her I'll be out in a second."

Something's wrong, I thought to myself. My mother never calls me during the day like this. Whatever she had to say, I knew it wasn't going to be good.

"Nance...." my mother said through her tears. "Eric is in the hospital. He was rushed to the emergency room this morning and they found a blood clot in his leg, but.....there's something else...they x-rayed him.....all over his body. Nancy, he's full of cancer. In his testicles, in his kidneys and in his lungs...." And then my mother started to cry like I've never heard her cry before.

Suddenly, I couldn't stand. I felt a wave of heat rush over my whole body as I tried to find the nearest seat.

"Okay, Mom, I'll be down as soon as I can. Don't drive anywhere. Just stay put."

The next hour was a blur.

Jeff got me into the car and we were on our way to the hospital. A heavy rain began to fall. The afternoon commute was bad, but my mind was solely on my younger brother Eric, only 42 years old, who married his job instead of a girlfriend and never had any kids. My two children were like his own. How were they going to take this news? What if he couldn't fight this? What if it was too late to help him?

Testicular cancer. It had spread all over his body. I could hear Jeff saying something about how Lance Armstrong had testicular cancer and it spread all over his body too – and he beat it. That's good, I thought to myself. But I bet Lance Armstrong didn't smoke a pack of cigarettes every day, nor did he know all the guys at the local pizza place on a first name basis.

We had a big battle ahead of us.

At the hospital, I knocked lightly on the heavy wooden door and slowly walked through.
"Hi." I said softly. "How are you feeling?"

My brother was lying in his bed. Suddenly, his eyes popped open. "Hey....did mom tell you? It's testicular cancer."

"Yes." I said. "Where's mom?"

"Trying to find something to eat in the cafeteria. They're going to remove the tumor tomorrow morning. They don't know about the other spots yet. Then start chemo soon afterwards." he said.

"Okay." I said. "You're going to be alright." The look in his eyes told me he didn't believe me.

"You know...I will help you fight this every single step of the way. I will take you to the best doctors in the country if I have to. Lance Armstrong beat this and you will too." I said, trying not to cry.

He nodded his head.

My mother returned to the room and we stayed with him for the next half hour making small talk. Then I walked over to his bed to kiss him goodbye.

"I'll see you tomorrow. I love you." I said. Those three words – I love you. Nobody in my family ever said them except for myself and my grandmother when she was alive.

I turned towards the door and slowly walked out.

"Nance?" Eric said.

"Yeah?" I said as I turned around.

"I love you, too."

Chapter Two
Fight with Everything You've Got

Eric's surgery was successful.

He would eventually follow it up with 1-week rounds of chemotherapy carried out every four weeks for four consecutive months. But he would never get around to starting his last round of chemo (more on that later), and suffered from everything from cachexia (severe muscle wasting) to pneumonia and depression.

I stayed true to my word and was there to support him every day. And at night, after putting the kids to bed, I would jump online and devour all the information I could find on his condition. The health research and medical sleuthing wasn't foreign to me. I had been doing it for myself and others almost as a part-time job since I suffered from postpartum depression after my daughter's birth in 2005. It prompted me to open a wellness center in 2006. I loved to solve health problems and Eric needed all the help he could get.

Cancer is a systemic disease. It has intelligence. It can adapt. It takes a lot more than the conventional cancer-killing methods to get the upper hand in the long run. Please understand, I am not trying to deter you from using any of the conventional methods in any way. You need a doctor. But there must be multiple layers of support if the enemy is to be defeated. Some of those layers may come from alternative methods of healing.

When a country goes to war, the leader doesn't just send in the infantry to attack the enemy for a few months and then call it quits. The leader sends in the best land and sea vehicles, and the best fighter pilots. They send in the spies and the special ops with the best satellite-backed technology in the world.

This is how to fight cancer. From all directions. You fight with everything you've got.

My brother smoked a pack of cigarettes every day. He never ate anything green on his own free will. He had no wife or kids to live for, just a pain-in-the-ass sister and two nagging parents, (although he does have another sister, but she lives too far away). Maybe he would live for my children, who knows. He was being pumped full of poisonous chemotherapy every month. He desperately needed something to support his healthy cells that were trying to survive the malaise of chaos unleashed in his body.

And then I found the support he would need – **through essential oils**.

Chapter Three
The Cancer-Killing Power of Essential Oils

When I opened my wellness center ten years ago, we used essential oils in many of the facial, spa, and body treatments, mainly for detoxification and relaxation purposes. But it wasn't until after my brother's diagnoses that I began to look at them in a completely different light. A friend met me for dinner one night, mentioned essential oils as a way to help support my brother's immune system, and the rest, as they say, is history.

As I dug deeper into the research, the clinical trials, and the documented testimonials, I was completely amazed by the power of these oils to adapt and seek and destroy abnormal cells while leaving the normal and healthy cells unscathed.

Specifically, the work of two doctors – Dr. Mahmoud Suhail, an immunologist from Iraq and Dr. H.K. Lin, a professor of Urology at the University of Oklahoma – caught my attention for their work using the essential oils of two specific plant species to put test subjects into remission very quickly. Some cases within a few weeks with no signs of malignancy.

These two doctors, working together, have pinpointed a specific compound called "AKBA" that is able to trigger apoptosis in the malignant cells. And I was about to find out firsthand how to use it effectively. I'll will show you how to do the same.

What Exactly Are Essential Oils?

These are the oils extracted from the leaf, bark, root, flower, seed, sap or peel of a plant. They are literally part of the plant's immune system and each species of plant possesses its own unique blend of potent compounds. These compounds have healing potential and have been used by many civilizations for thousands of years to keep the general population safe and healthy.

Here are some amazing facts about essential oils:

- Each drop of essential oil has enough molecules to cover every cell in the human body 40,000 times.
- Each molecule of oil is so microscopic in size, they can pass through the epidermis and enter the bloodstream within minutes, and can even pass through the blood/brain barrier with ease. To give you an example, if you were to put one drop of peppermint essential oil on the bottom of your foot, you would be able to taste peppermint in your mouth within 10 minutes as the menthol and menthone rapidly spreads, touching every cell in your body.
- Essential oils carry the highest amount of oxygenating molecules of any substance known to man. This is key since cancer cells cannot thrive long-term in a consistently oxygenated environment.
- In addition to oxygen, these molecules also carry minerals, amino acids, and other vital nutrients to the cell.
- Essential oils stimulate secretagogues needed for producing hormones that heal the body.

Essential oils have three very important classes of compounds that are key in creating good health:

1. Phenols, which clean the cell walls including the hormone receptor sites so that proper communication between cells is improved. Examples of essential oils high in phenols would be clove and peppermint.
2. Sesquiterpenes, which have the ability to permeate the cell wall and deliver massive amounts of oxygen to the cell. They can also erase or deprogram misinformation within the DNA of an abnormal cell. Examples of essential oils high in sesquiterpenes would be cedarwood and sandalwood. Cedarwood oil is made up of 98% sesquiterpenes.
3. Monoterpenes, which have the ability to reprogram and correct misinformation within the DNA. Examples of oils that have high quantities of monoterpenes are frankincense and sacred frankincense.

Chapter Four
The Reset Button: Two Key Compounds That Create a One-Two Punch Against Cancer

In 1985, long before Dr. Suhail and H.K. Lin began their research, two professors from Brigham Young University, one professor from the Botany Department and the other from the Biochemistry Department were inspired by what they were seeing with the effects of essential oils on cancer and conducted their own studies on several cancer lines.

In their research, they tested 74 different essential oils – 69 single oils and the remaining 5 oils were blends – on skin cancer, cervical cancer, breast cancer, and prostate cancer. They used a mono-layer with various concentrations of each oil, saturated for a minimum 24-hour period and incubated at 37 degrees Celsius. The results were astounding and showed 58% of the oils demonstrated a general cancer kill rate of at least 50% or higher.

Here are some of the results that were seen:

Sandalwood essential oil was tested at a dilution of 100 parts per million and had a 97.2% effective kill rate on cervical cancer, an 84% kill rate on prostate cancer, a 98% kill rate on breast cancer, and a 58% rate on skin cancer.

Hyssop oil had a kill rate of 90% against cervical cancer and 75% against skin cancer.

Grapefruit essential oil had an 80% kill rate against skin

cancer cells. Thyme essential oil had an astounding 99% effective kill rate against cervical cancer. Amazing.

But the two plant species that exhibited an exceptionally high rate of DNA repair were frankincense and sandalwood. These two essential oils are used as the base of all cancer-fighting protocols.

What makes these oils so special?

Sandalwood oil is a sesquiterpene and frankincense is a monoterpene. Both have the ability to kill cancer on their own, but when they are used together synergistically, the cancer-killing effect is amplified because they attack cancer cells in two very different ways.

The sesquiterpene, alpha-santalol in sandalwood oil induces non-selective cell death by triggering a negative regulation of protein kinase activity. In other words, **the sandalwood oil can erase and deactivate abnormal information in the DNA.**

Frankincense, on the other hand, is made up of monoterpenes which have the ability to rewrite the misinformation in the DNA. It does this through the activation of histone proteins found in the eukaryotic cell nuclei that bind the DNA into nucleosomes. Frankincense is like a "reset" button in the DNA makeup.

So when you use the sandalwood, you are erasing the bad information and by using the frankincense you are replacing the bad information with good information in the DNA.

Frankincense also has a special compound in it called "AKBA." It is acetyl-11-keto-beta boswellic acid and it is so powerful, it has the ability to adapt and destroy cancer cells that chemotherapy can't touch. It literally penetrates the malignant cell wall and disconnects the nucleus from the rest of the cell.

These essential oils have proteins in them and proteins have intelligence. Think of what a smart bomb is and what it is capable of doing. It targets and destroys only where you need it and does not destroy the areas where you don't need it. This is what the AKBA compound can do for cancer as well.

Most Extraordinary Cancer Cases

Professor of Urology, H.K. Lin, describes in an interview, some of the most fascinating examples of healing he has seen using essential oils in research studies, including a stage 4 breast cancer patient whom doctors had given up on.

> *"After using frankincense therapeutically, the primary tumor, which was 9.5 x 12.5 x 11 cm's, in the left breast began the process of necrosis and started shedding off for a period of 5-8 weeks, leaving only a tiny malignant ulcer. The secondary metastatic lesions on the patient's body just shrank and disappeared."*

Dr. Lin also describes a terminal patient who suffered from adenocarcinoma which is a cancer that forms in mucus-secreting glands and is prevalent in lung, prostate, colorectal, and pancreatic cancers.

> *"A primary lesion in the ascending colon metastasized to the liver and hepatobiliary tract, with some peritoneal foci of metastasis ascites, lymph nodes, and peri-aortic lymph nodes. The carcinoembryonic antigen was 210 International Units per millimeter. (The normal range is 5-10 IU's)*

When it is more than 10, it is a high probability of cancer presence, and if it is more than 20 it is metastasis for sure.

In this case, carcinoembryonic antigen declined from 210 to 18 in exactly 16 days.

The metastatic foci disappeared in 21 days and the primary tumor underwent necrosis and shrunk in size to disappear in an additional 3-4 weeks."

But before you rush out to your local health food store and buy up all the essential oils in their inventory, there is one thing you need to be aware of. You need the right essential oils, and those oils are not what you would find at the store.

Not All Essential Oils Are Made the Same Way

The majority of essential oils are extracted using the steam distillation method. There are a few exceptions though, most citrus oils are cold-pressed. However, lime essential oil is usually steam distilled because the skin can be too leathery to press.

The quality of an essential oil depends on many things – how long the oil is distilled, the temperature, and even what time of year the plant is harvested matters when it comes to producing quality.

According to Dr. Suhail, frankincense essential oil needs to be distilled for a minimum of at least 12 hours at 100 degrees Celsius for the presence of cancer-killing compounds to rise dramatically. Anything less is not up to standard and may not produce the desired results.

There are four grades of essential oils: Grade A, or therapeutic grade oil, Grade B, or food grade oil, Grade C - fragrance grade, and Grade D - floral water.

What you are looking for is Grade A therapeutic essential oil. However, many of the therapeutic oils sold in health food stores are not pure and have been cut with synthetic extenders. The retail price is a tell-tale sign. The high quality frankincense cannot be purchased for under $55 per 15 ml. bottle. Anything less than that and you are purchasing an inferior product.

The FDA prohibits me from mentioning the brand that I have used, but if you Google "essential oils company Lehi Utah" you should find the correct source. Essential oils from this source are believed to be safe for taking internally.

Chapter Five
How to Use Essential Oils Effectively

We were having the coldest winter in years. I looked at the latest weather report - two feet of snow in the next forty-eight hours and blizzard conditions. We were hunkered down and ready to ride the storm out. I looked at the clock on the wall – 10:45 p.m. Time to get to bed.

Then I heard the phone ring.

"Mom? What's going on?" I said.

"Eric. I think we're losing him." she said.

Eric was near the end of his third round of chemotherapy and not doing well. He was not taking his supplements like the doctor had ordered. He stopped eating. To deal with the constant pain and nausea, he was still smoking cigarettes – something the doctor assured me he would lose interest in once he started his chemo. Because of the smoking and the chemotherapy, he developed pneumonia. His weight dwindled down to 135 lbs. which hung on his 6' 1" frame.

"Okay, Mom. Keep the lights on for me. I'll be there in an hour."

I had not given him very much of the essential oils at that point because I was worried it would interfere with his medication.

The latest scan indicated that the cancer was dying – but so was everything else in his body – except for a spot on his left lung. It was not getting smaller. It was growing. And now his kidneys were shutting down.

I climbed the stairs which led to his bedroom and found him lying in the fetal position – a shadow of the person he once was, only a few months ago. I tried to hide my tears.

"Eric? It's me. Why aren't you trying to eat? Why aren't you listening to the doctor?" I waited for the answer but the answer never came.

"You know what?" I said, "You are GOING to start listening. You are GOING to stop smoking. And you are GOING to live, Do you hear me? You want to give up and die? I don't think so. Because I'll be damned if I'm going to sit here and watch my children lose their favorite uncle because you gave up! And you are NOT leaving me here alone to take care of Mom and Dad. That is not NOT happening!"

Eric's eyes slowly opened. He was too weak to tell me to go to hell, or to even care. He just nodded his head.

"I'm going to start using these essential oils on you. We're going to hit it hard. Okay?" I said.

He nodded his head again.

"Okay."

I left the room and went downstairs to talk to my mother. We were stuck between a rock and a hard place. There was still a spot of malignant cells growing in Eric's left lung, but because he wasn't doing the things he was ordered to do, he had to stop the chemotherapy or risk dying from organ failure.

It was time to use Plan B.

It was time to start applying the essential oils.

How to Do the Oils Application

You are going to apply the oils every day for 21 days as directed and then check your markers for improvement.

There are three (3) places where the oils are applied:

- the spine
- the bottoms of the feet
- the tumor site(s) if possible

You will need a loved one to help massage the oils into the spine and the feet. The spine massage is given at least once per day and the foot application is given at least once per day. Application to the tumor site is done every four to five hours.

In each application you are using only a few drops of oil.

Each type of cancer has its own special list of oils that work best. I have gone ahead and listed them out in the next chapter. If you cannot find your type of cancer listed, you can use the Basic Procedure.

But every application must start with a sesquiterpene and a monoterpene. Frankincense or Sacred Frankincense as your monoterpene, and Sandalwood or Cedarwood as your sesquiterpene. Always.

The Basic Procedure:
Use these essentials oils for the spine and foot massages. Do at least one of each massage every day for 21 days and then have markers checked. Don't do both massages at the same time. Space them out at least 8 hours apart from each other.

Once you apply the essential oils to the skin, the compounds stay in your system for approximately 3-4 hours, so you want to space out the applications. Remember, in addition to the spine and foot massages you will also be applying the oils to the tumor/cancer site and will also be ingesting some of the oils, so there will be a continuous presence of cancer-killing compounds in the body as much as possible.

For the Basic Procedure, use:
- Frankincense
- Sandalwood
- Cedarwood
- Idaho Balsam Fir
- Copaiba (pronounced KO-pah-EE-bah) for pain

For the spine massage, start with your sesquiterpene – either Sandalwood or Cedarwood. (If cost is an issue, you can use more of the Cedarwood. I refer to Cedarwood as the "poor man's Sandalwood" because it costs a fraction of what the Sandalwood costs and it actually has more sesquiterpenes in it than the Sandalwood).

Drop approximately 5 drops of Cedarwood down the back, starting from the back of the neck and put one drop down the spine every 5 inches or so, ending at the top of the buttocks close to the tailbone.

Massage with the fingertips with both hands moving the

fingertips in small clockwise circles on top of the spine, starting behind the neck and massaging down ending at the top of the buttocks.

Repeat the process with the Sandalwood.

Repeat the process with the Frankincense.

Repeat with Idaho Balsam Fir.

End with Copaiba.

Copaiba essential oil is actually a sap taken from the female copaiba tree from South America and it's used for pain management and it also intensifies the other oils that were massaged into the spine before it. Always put this on last.

Don't mix the oils together in an effort to save time. The oils must be applied in a layered fashion. The act of massage itself, is a method which stimulates the immune system. So try to relax and enjoy being cared for.

Foot Massage

Hold the bottle of essential oil in your left hand and place a drop in your right hand. Then with your oily hand you are going to swipe the bottom of the foot from heel to toes so that you cover the bottom of the foot with the oil.

Next, hold the foot with both hands and massage the bottom of the foot with your thumbs in small circular motions using medium pressure. If you'd like, you can use foot reflexology or something called Vita Flex to massage specific points on the bottom of the feet. Each section – toes, heel, ball of the foot –

correlates with part of the body. You can easily google "Vita Flex Foot Chart" and it will show you.

I usually just massage the entire foot with my thumbs starting on each toe and then working down to the heel.

Start with your sesquiterpenes like you did with the spine massage, then do your monoterpene (Frankincense) and end with the other oils.

Apply Oils at the Tumor Site

For this step, you are going to rub one drop of each of the oils into the tumor area. If you can't touch the tumor area, get as close as you can to it. Do this every 4 or 5 hours.

Taking the Oils by Mouth

For this part of the application, you will use only Frankincense, Idaho Balsam Fir, and Copaiba. Go to your local health food store and buy empty veggie capsules. Fill one capsule with 3 drops of each of the oils. Take this with a little bit of food every 6 hours or so.

This blend is used to manage pain. If you are in greater pain you may take these capsules every 3-4 hours instead.

Putting It All Together

You may want to start the day by getting a spine massage and then taking some of the oils by mouth. Then a couple hours later, apply the oils to the tumor site. A few hours later, take the oils by mouth again and then afterwards apply to the tumor site. Continue this until evening when you end the day with the foot massage. You will get some overlap with the applications and that is perfectly fine. The point is to keep the cells bathed in the compounds constantly.

After the 21 days of essential oils therapy, you want to "test and rest." Go back to your doctor and look at your progress. You will also take a break from the oils for about a week.

Then you will start another 21 day cycle using essential oils, but here is where you will switch things up a bit.

Confusing the Cancer Cells

At this point, you will switch things around a little to confuse the malignant cells. Keep using Frankincense and Cedarwood in the basic mix, but instead of the other oils, you will be using some citrus oils.

(Please note: If you have liver cancer, your first 21 days of application of oils calls for some citrus oils already, so for your second 21 day stretch you should use the Basic Procedure oils instead to confuse the cancer cells).

Citrus essential oils do a few things, but most importantly, they increase the amount of glutathione in the body. Glutathione is a powerful guardian of your health and it's also referred to as "the mother of all antioxidants." Increasing it will help rebuild cells that have been damaged and usher out the cells that cannot be repaired.

Citrus oils also brighten your mood and can lift you out of depression. Studies have proven that just by inhaling a bit of orange, the olfactory system triggers feelings of happiness and orange can make you feel less irritated, angry, and hopeless.

Part Two of Essential Oils Application

Remember, you are going to do this for a 21 day cycle after taking a one-week break from the first procedure.

Use these essential oils:

- Frankincense
- Cedarwood
- Orange
- Lemon
- Tangerine

Follow the same instructions for the spine and foot massages using these oils. For the capsule, you should still use the Frankincense, Idaho Balsam Fir, and the Copaiba and take as before.

After you have completed these 21 days, you should test and rest again. Measure your progress and then go back to the original procedure for the next 21-day cycle if necessary.

Procedure for Different Types of Cancer

Through research it has been discovered that certain essential oils work better and differently on specific types of cancer. I have listed several types of cancer below, and which oils work the best on them.

Remember to always use your sesquiterpenes and monoterpenes first and then apply the other oils in layers when doing your spine and foot massages, just like you would do with the Basic Procedure. If you can't find your particular cancer listed below, just use the Basic Procedure instructions.

Also, for the capsules, always use the blend of Frankincense, Idaho Balsam Fir, and Copaiba no matter which kind of cancer you are dealing with.

Bone Cancer

- Frankincense
- Sandalwood
- Cedarwood
- Clove
- Tsuga
- Idaho Balsam Fir
- Copaiba

Please note: Clove oil is a very "hot" oil and should only be used on the bottom of the feet and not on the back or directly on the tumor site as it will create discomfort on the skin. Again, it is perfectly safe for the bottom of the foot.

If you accidentally get Clove oil on the skin and it causes discomfort, apply any kind of carrier oil such as coconut oil or even olive oil to the area to sooth the skin. NEVER try to wash the essential oil off of the skin with water. Water will drive the oil deeper into the skin and will cause the discomfort to intensify.

Breast Cancer

- Sacred Frankincense
- Sandalwood
- Cedarwood
- Idaho Balsam Fir
- Myrtle
- Copaiba

One word of caution: If you are taking Tamoxifen for breast cancer, do not apply citrus essential oils to your body. You may use the other oils listed in your second course of applications, but skip the use of citrus oils.

Cervical Cancer

- Frankincense
- Sandalwood
- Idaho Balsam Fir
- Patchouli
- Hyssop
- Tarragon
- Copaiba
- Thyme

Colon Cancer

- Frankincense
- Sandalwood
- Idaho Balsam Fir
- Clove
- Ledum
- Tsuga
- Lavender
- Copaiba

Again, Clove oil is to be used only on the bottom of the feet.

Hodgkin's Disease

- Frankincense
- Sandalwood
- Clove
- Lavender
- Cistus
- Idaho Balsam Fir
- Copaiba

Leukemia

- Frankincense
- Sandalwood
- Cedarwood
- Clove
- Lavender
- Idaho Balsam Fir
- Copaiba

Liver Cancer

- Frankincense
- Sandalwood
- Cedarwood
- Orange
- Lemon
- Thyme
- Idaho Balsam Fir
- Copaiba

Lung Cancer

- Frankincense
- Cedarwood
- Orange
- Thyme
- Sage
- Idaho Balsam Fir
- Copaiba
- Ravensara

Skin Cancer

- Frankincense
- Sandalwood
- Helichrysum
- Grapefruit
- Tarragon
- Idaho Balsam Fir
- Copaiba

Ovarian Cancer

- Sacred Frankincense
- Sandalwood
- Cypress
- Myrrh
- Geranium
- Idaho Balsam Fir
- Copaiba

Prostate Cancer

- Frankincense
- Cedarwood
- Sandalwood
- Thyme
- Myrtle
- Idaho Balsam Fir
- Copaiba

Chapter Six
Remission

After failure to complete the required rounds of chemotherapy, the spot on Eric's lung was still thriving, and we felt we needed a second opinion to see what his next move would be. I had taken over his care and we hit the cancer hard with the essential oils. About 5 weeks later, the new oncologist in Boston accepted our request for a visit and had my brother submit to a whole new round of tests. Approximately two weeks after that, Eric's new doctor summoned him to his office at the Yawkey Building at Mass General Hospital.

I was a wreck sitting in the waiting room.

Prior to coming to the appointment, the doctor explained to Eric what his choices might be depending on what the results of the scan were. Surgery or more chemotherapy. Both had serious life-threatening ramifications.

"Please God." I said to myself. "Just give me a few more weeks with the oils. That's all I'm asking. Just a little more time so they can work."

"Eric?" the nurse called out into the waiting area. "Come this way, please."

We got up and slowly made our way to the back office area.

We sat in the examination room for what seemed like forever, and then in came the new doctor – a smile on his face.

"Hi Eric. I'm Dr. Michaelson, how are you doing?"

We made the usual nervous small talk.

"Well, Eric, I looked at the pictures of your lung and there's a problem. It's a very good problem, though. I can't seem to find any evidence that you have cancer!" he said.

"Wait. What?" I said in disbelief.

"We can't find any cancer in your brother. None."

I let out a cry of relief and the tears began to flow.

"We'll keep an eye on it and if there is no sign of the cancer coming back in the next 2 to 3 years, I would say you will be in great shape going forward. Congratulations!"

Since putting cancer into remission, Eric works to make his body an inhospitable place for cancer to thrive.

He continues to use Frankincense every day and rubs several drops into his chest along with a few drops of Orange essential oil to keep his glutathione levels up.

I give him one spine and one foot massage per month using the oils in the Basic Protocol.

An addition to the oils, he also takes 10,000 IU's of Vitamin D3 with 300mcg's of Vitamin K2 and keeps his Vitamin D serum levels above 50 ng/ml.

Keeping your serum levels between 50 ng/ml and 100 ng/ml is a great way to deter cancer for the long haul – just make sure it's Vitamin D3, not D2. D3 is easier for your body to use and it's more potent than D2. Have your doctor or health care provider check your levels every few months to make sure you don't go over 100 ng/ml or under 40 ng/ml and you'll be in good shape.

I wish you nothing but great health and success in your journey!

Please look for my second book coming soon:

**Essential Oils and Cancer:
How to Create Creams,
Cleansers, and Deodorants
That Protect the Immune System**

References

"Cancer Hope" Ammon H.P. Boswellic acid in chronic inflammatory diseases. Planta Med 2006; 72 (12): 1100-16

Khajuria A. et al Immunomodulatory activity of biopolymeric fraction BOS 2000 from Boswellia serrata. Phytother Res 2008; 22(3): 340-8.

Kirste S, et al. Boswellia serrata acts on cerebral edema in patients irradiated for brain tumors: a prospective, randomized, placebo-controlled, double-blind pilot trial. Cancer 2011; 117 (16): 3788-95

Park B, et al. Boswellic acid suppresses growth and metastasis of human pancreatic tumors in an orthotopic mouse model through modulation of multiple targets. PloS One. 2011; 6(10): e26943 [epub]

Suhail MM, et al. Boswellia sacra essential oil induces tumor cell-specific apoptosis and suppresses tumor aggressiveness in cultured human breast cancer cells. BMC Complement Altern Med 2011; 11:129.

Takahashi M. et al. Boswellic acid exerts anti-tumor effects in colorectal cancer cells by modulating expression of the let-7 and miR-200 microRNA family. Carcinogenesis 2012; 33(12): 2441-9.

Yuan Y, et al. Acetyl-11-keto-beta-boswellic acid (AKBA) prevents human colonic adenocarcinoma growth through modulation of multiple signaling pathways. Biochim Biophys Acta 2013; 1830(10): 4907-16.

Zhang YS, et al. Acetyl-11-keto-beta- boswellic acid (AKBA) inhibits human gastric carcinoma growth through modulation of the Wnt/beta-catenin signaling pathway. Biochim Biophys Acta 2013; 1830(6): 3604-15.

http://www.ncbi.nlm.nih.gov/pubmedhealth/behindtheheadlines/news/2013-12-23-can-frankincense-really-fight-cancer/23Dec2013

http://theresanoilforthat.blogspot.com/2012/02/frankincenseandcancer.html

http://www.dailymail.co.uk/health/article-2526816/Frankincense-fights-cancer-Aromatic-substance-Nativity-story-help-treat-ovarian-tumours.html

http://gulfnews.com/news/gulf/oman/oman-researchers-find-cancer-treatment-in-frankincense-1.1251940

http://ecancer.org/news/465.php

"Frankincense Oil – A Potential Treatment Option for Bladder Cancer"

"Differential effects of selective frankincense essential oil versus non-selective sandalwood essential oil on cultured bladder cancer cells: a microarray and bioinformatics study" Mikhail G Dozmorov, Qing Yang, Weijuan Wu, Jonathan Wren, Mahmoud M Suhail, Cole Wooley, D Gary Young, Kar-Ming Fung, and Hsueh-Kung Lin
Corresponding author: HK Lin
Chinese Medicine 2014, 9:18
http://www.cmjournal.org/content/9/1/18

Made in the USA
Columbia, SC
24 May 2020

98252900R00026